THE ARTHRITIS DIET

Anti-Inflammatory Diet Foods for
Beginners to Reduce Joint Inflammation
and Relieve Arthritis Pain

Nancy Peterson

TABLE OF CONTENT

3

Introduction

It can be very devastating to be diagnosed with arthritis. Arthritis is a general term for conditions that cause chronic inflammation and joint pain. Arthritis is known to cause swelling, pain and joint stiffness. It is not peculiar to any age as it can happen to anybody, any ethnic background and all genders. There are several types of arthritis which includes osteoarthritis, rheumatoid arthritis (which is an autoimmune disease that makes your immune system to attack your joints) and psoriatic arthritis. The typical treatment for arthritis involves pain and inflammation reducing medications.

However, its consoling to know that there are several foods that you can eat to relieve inflammation and joint pains associated with arthritis. In fact, from one survey conducted, 24% of people with rheumatoid arthritis confirmed that their symptoms reduced drastically when they changed what they eat.

Inflammation is natural as it aids the body to heal and defend itself against harm. Inflammation helps the body to protect itself from injury, illness and infection. In response to inflammation, your body begins to increase the amount of white blood cells it produces along with increased production of immune cells and cytokines that helps to fight infections. However, when inflammation becomes chronic, it then becomes harmful to the body.

Some signs of acute inflammation include pain, swelling, redness and heat for short term inflammation. While the chronic, long term inflammation can happen in your body without showing any identifiable symptoms. This type of inflammation can cause heart disease, diabetes, cancer and fatty liver disease.

How Does Change in Diet Help with Arthritis

Although we do not have exact diets or dietary supplements that can totally cure your arthritis, however, several people have testified that they witnessed an improvement in their symptoms when they changed what they eat. Let us also bear in mind that we are all different and there are also many types of arthritis, based on this, what may work for a certain type of arthritis or what may work for you may not work for the other. But research has found several connections between one's diet and arthritis, so it is important to consider what you eat when treating arthritis.

Changing your diet alone would not be as impactful except if you combine with exercise and your medical treatment. It is important that you confirm from your doctor before you stop taking your medical prescriptions.

The two most important things you should note when treating arthritis are:

- **Your weight:** if you are overweight, it would be beneficial to lose some weights so as to reduce strain on your joints. Once you are able to achieve this, you would no longer need to depend on painkillers as often as you do now.

- **Your diet:** Asides your diet equipping you with the needed minerals and vitamins, a good diet is also helpful in protecting one against some potential side effect of drugs. The right diet also fights against heart disease which can arise as one of the complication that patients face when treating some types of arthritis.

Some types of arthritis and the drugs for treatment have been confirmed to cause an increased risk in circulatory and heart problems. Several changes in diets and lifestyles that benefits patients with arthritis are also beneficial for heart and circulatory health like the omega-3 fatty acids and exercise.

No matter the type of arthritis that you have been diagnosed with, you should ensure to eat:

- A varied and balanced diet to give you all the antioxidants, minerals, vitamins and other nutrients that your body needs.
- More of the Mediterranean style diet that includes pulses, olive oil, fish and plenty of vegetables and fruits.
- Consume more of foods rich in omega-3 fatty acids which can be gotten from oily fish for instance.
- Ensure to exercise regularly.

Anti-Inflammatory Diet for Arthritis

An anti-inflammatory diet helps to reduce chronic pain caused by rheumatoid arthritis, osteoarthritis and other types of inflammatory arthritis like the ankylosing spondylitis and the psoriatic arthritis.

An example of the anti-inflammatory diet is the well-known Mediterranean diet. An anti-inflammatory diet does not encourage the consumption of processed foods while it supports eating of beans, vegetables, whole grains, fruits and foods that have omega-3 fatty acids like the wild salmon and the anchovies in oil. Apart from being able to reduce chronic arthritis pains, the anti-inflammatory diet also helps to promote long term health.

Understanding the Anti-inflammatory Diet

Consuming anti-inflammatory foods would not only reduce pains from arthritis but would also benefit the overall health in a long-term basis. It is very important for you to know the foods that promote and prevent inflammation. It is also important that you understand the points below:

- An anti-inflammatory diet is not just a short-term solution but a total change of lifestyle.
- The anti-inflammatory diet is not same for everyone and can vary from one person to the other depending on an individual's biology.
- Exercise also helps to improve the positive effects of the anti-inflammatory diet for treating arthritis pains.
- Anti-inflammatory Diet is not One Size Fits All.
- Research have shown that some types of diet would work better for certain individuals than another just like medications. For example: Some people experience reduced pain and

inflammation when they eliminate some certain foods that causes inflammation for them. For instance, while the whole wheat is considered a healthy meal, some people however discover that gluten, which is made from proteins found in wheat, helps to encourage inflammation in their system.

- While one person may experience a notable reduction in arthritis pain and inflammation when on the traditional anti-inflammatory diet, another person may have little or no positive effect from the diet.

Because of this, it is important to work with your nutritionist or doctor to experiment with different foods until you find the one that would soothe your arthritis pain.

How Foods Help to Suppress Arthritis Inflammation

While inflammation is important to the human immune systems, ironically, it is also the root cause of most pains associated with arthritis. Also, as people grow older, their metabolism change and they become more prone to inflammation even when they are not injured or sick. Certain foods are known to worsen these inflammatory conditions.

To help you understand the role foods play in suppressing arthritis inflammation or how these foods can cause inflammation, it is important that you understand what oxidative stress, free radicals and antioxidants mean.

- **Free radicals:** sometimes called reactive oxygen species, are negatively charged molecules or atoms. Free radicals by nature, search for other positively charged molecules or atoms to bond with (oxidation). The body helps to create free radicals as part of its normal metabolism; however, the body can produce too many free radicals when exposed to some behavioral factors like consuming some types of food or smoking.

- **Oxidative stress:** While the body is known to naturally neutralize and process these free radicals, however, when they become too many, the body system would become overwhelmed and thereby create an imbalance. This imbalance is referred to as oxidative stress.

- **Inflammation:** Oxidative stress can lead to chronic inflammation. Many experts are of the opinion that oxidative stress starts a biochemical cascade that encourages inflammation and can overtime lead to related degenerative diseases like the arthritis.

- **Antioxidants:** Antioxidants trap and neutralize free radicals. Antioxidants are either produced from within the body or gotten from foods that we eat as well as anti-inflammatory drugs we take.

An anti-inflammatory diet helps to eliminate or cut down foods that can cause oxidative stress while encouraging the consumption of foods that are rich in antioxidants. The aim of the anti-inflammatory diet for arthritis is to lower unnecessary inflammations and the pain and joint degeneration that it may cause.

Understanding Fatty Acids

Our body's digestive system helps to break down the fats and oils we eat into fatty acids. However, the body cannot produce other fatty acids and they can only be gotten from foods, these ones are called the essential fatty acids (EFAs). There are two groups of polyunsaturated fatty acids; omega-3 and omega-6.

The omega-3 fatty acids are in two forms:

- Short-chain forms found in flaxseed oil, rapeseed oil and walnuts.
- Long chain forms found in higher levels in oily fish. Examples are sardines, pilchards, salmon and mackerel.

Omega-3 have been proven to help people that have the inflammatory types of arthritis like the reactive arthritis, rheumatoid arthritis, ankylosing and psoriatic arthritis.

Anti-inflammatory Foods

Many foods have natural chemical compounds that have anti-inflammatory properties, examples of these foods are vegetables and fruits. The foods listed below are highly recommended on our list of anti-inflammatory foods:

- Certain spices like turmeric and ginger.
- Cold water fish like salmon, tuna, bass, mackerel, anchovies and sardines
- Green tea and water especially mineral water.
- Fresh and frozen foods like apricots, apples, berries, bananas, kiwi fruit, avocados, pineapples, grapes, papaya, cantaloupe and oranges.
- Chia seeds, flaxseeds and tofu.
- Whole grains including rice, wheat, quinoa, spelt, oats, millet, bulgur wheat, buckwheat and barley.
- Certain oils including olive oils and flaxseed.
- Nuts including walnuts, almonds and macadamia nuts

- Deep green vegetables like the kale, spinach, collards, swiss chard and broccoli.
- Other vegetables like carrots, celery, cabbage, onions, sweet potatoes and cauliflower.

Vegetable oils, fish, flaxseed oil, walnuts, chia seeds, flax seeds and leafy vegetables in particular are rich in omega-3 fatty acids. Evidence from scientific research shows that diets rich in omega-3 fatty acids can cause a modest reduction of symptoms in rheumatoid arthritis patients.

Best Foods to Eat with Arthritis

Fatty Fish

Fatty fish variance like mackerel, trout, sardines and salmon are rich in omega-3 fatty acids that have been proven to have powerful anti-inflammatory effects.

In a small study conducted, 33 participants were fed either lean meat, fatty fish or lean fish four times every week. At the end of 8 weeks, the group that were fed with fatty acids experienced a decrease in the levels of specific compounds that causes inflammation.

Another analysis of 17 different studies confirmed that when you take omega 3 fatty acid supplements, it would help to reduce the intensity of joint pain, number of painful joints and morning stiffness. This would also cause a reduced use of pain relief medicines when treating rheumatoid arthritis.

Another test tube study also showed that omega-3 fatty acids helps to reduce several inflammatory markers found in osteoarthritis.

Fish is also rich in vitamin D to help prevent deficiency. Several studies proved that rheumatoid arthritis may be linked with reduced levels of vitamin D, that can contribute to symptoms.

The American Heart Association advises that you include at least two servings of fatty fish in your diet every week to enjoy its beneficial anti-inflammatory properties.

Garlic

Garlic has a lot of health benefits. Several test tube studies show that garlic helps to fight cancer. It is also rich in compounds that may help to reduce your risk of having dementia and heart disease.

Also, studies have proven that garlic has anti-inflammatory effects that plays a great role in reducing symptoms of arthritis. From research, we are made to know that garlic can improve the functions of specific immune cells to help make the immune system stronger.

In one study carried out by researchers, the diets of 1,082 twins were analyzed and it was discovered that participants who ate more garlic had a lowered risk of hip osteoarthritis likely because of the strong anti-inflammatory properties found in garlic. A similar test tube study conducted showed that some certain components found in garlic can reduce some of the things that cause inflammations that would ultimately lead to arthritis.

Adding garlic to your diet would not only benefit people with arthritis symptoms but is also beneficial to your overall health.

Ginger

Apart from its flavorful taste it gives to soups, teas and sweet, ginger also helps to relieve symptoms of arthritis.

A study conducted in 2001 evaluated the effects that ginger had on 261 patients that had knee osteoarthritis. After six weeks of consuming ginger in their meals, 63% of the participants felt an improvement with the knee pain.

Another tube test study conducted proved that ginger and its components help to block the body's production of substances that encourage inflammation in the human body. Yet another study conducted with rats showed that treating rats with extracts of ginger caused a decreased level of specific inflammatory market associated with arthritis.

Whether you consume ginger in its dried, powdered or fresh form, it would help to lower inflammation and also reduce symptoms of arthritis.

Broccoli

It is no longer news that broccoli is one of the healthiest foods we have on the planet. In fact, it has been linked with reduced inflammation.

One study that analyzed the diets of 1,005 women discovered that those who ate cruciferous vegetables like broccoli had a decreased level of inflammation symptoms.

Broccoli also have important components that can help to reduce symptoms of arthritis. For instance, sulforaphane is one of the compounds found in broccoli. From test tube studies conducted, we discovered that sulforaphane blocks the formation of a cell type linked with the development of rheumatoid arthritis.

Another study carried out with animals found that sulforaphane can help to reduce the production of some specific inflammatory markers that contributes to rheumatoid arthritis.

Although we may need more studies done with human, however, these animal studies and test tube studies have helped to prove that the compounds in broccoli is beneficial in reducing symptoms of arthritis.

Walnuts

This fruit is nutrient dense and also very rich in compounds that can help to reduce inflammation linked to joint disease.

13 studies were analyzed and it was discovered that when you eat walnuts, it helps to reduce symptoms that cause inflammation. Walnuts is very rich in omega-3 fatty acids which have been proved over time to reduce symptoms of arthritis.

In one study conducted, 90 patients that had rheumatoid arthritis were given supplements of either olive oil or omega-3 fatty acids. Those who took the omega-3 fatty acids experienced reduced pain levels than those who took the olive oil and they were able to reduce the frequency at which they use their arthritis medications.

Berries

Each servings of berries are packed with tons of vitamins, antioxidants and minerals which may be partly the reason for the fruit's unique ability to reduce inflammation. In one study that involved 38,176 women, participants who consumed at least two servings of strawberries every week had 14% less chances of having elevated level of inflammatory markers in the blood.

Also, berries have high content of rutin and quercetin, two great plant compounds that are very beneficial to your body health. From one test tube study conducted, it was discovered quercetin blocks some inflammatory processes that are associated with arthritis.

Fortunately, we have a wide option of berries to choose from to enjoy the massive health benefits of the berries. We have the blueberries, blackberries and strawberries to mention but a few, that can not only provide your body with plenty nutrients to fight arthritis, but would also satisfy your sweet tooth.

Spinach

Leafy greens like spinach contain several beneficial nutrients and some of its components are known to help reduce inflammation from arthritis. Several studies showed that when you increase your intake of vegetables and fruits, it would lead to reduced levels of inflammation. Spinach especially have plenty antioxidants and plant compounds that helps to soothe inflammation and fight diseases.

This vegetable is very high in antioxidant kaempferol, which has been proven to reduce the effects of agents of inflammation linked with rheumatoid arthritis. In a test tube study conducted in 2017, patients with arthritic cartilage cells were treated with the kaempferol and they experienced reduced inflammation and it also helped to prevent the osteoarthritis from progressing.

Grapes

Grapes are rich in antioxidants, nutrient-dense and also contains anti-inflammatory properties. In one study conducted, 24 men were given either a placebo or a concentrated grape powder that is equivalent to approximately 1 and half cups of fresh grapes daily for 3 weeks. The men who took the grape powder noticed an effective decrease in the levels of inflammatory markers in their blood.

Also, grapes have several compounds that are beneficial when treating arthritis. For instance, resveratrol is one antioxidant that is found in the skin of grapes. In a test tube study conducted, it was discovered that resveratrol has potential to help prevent the thickening of the joints connected with arthritis by blocking rheumatoid arthritis cells from forming.

Grapes also have a plant compound known as proanthocyanidin, which have promising impacts on arthritis. For instance, one test tube study showed that the proanthocyanidin extract from grape seed helped to reduce inflammation related to arthritis. However, bear in mind that these test tube studies make use of concentrated doses of antioxidants that are far more than the amount you would consume in a normal serving.

Olive oil

This is popularly known for its anti-inflammatory properties that are beneficial in soothing arthritis symptoms.

In a study conducted with mice, the mice were fed with extra virgin oil for 6 weeks. This helped to stop arthritis from developing, slowed the destruction of the cartilage, reduced swelling of the joints and also reduced inflammation.

Another study fed its 49 rheumatoid arthritis patients with either olive oil or fish oil capsule daily for 24 weeks. At the close of the study, each group experienced a reduced level of certain inflammatory markers; about 40 to 55% for those that took the fish oil and 38.5% for those that took the olive oil.

Another study looked at the diets of its 333 participants mixed with rheumatoid and non-rheumatoid arthritis patients and it was discovered that consuming olive oil helps to reduce risk of rheumatoid arthritis.

Adding the olive oil as well as other healthy fats in your diet would be a great benefit to your health as well as help to limit the symptoms of arthritis.

Tart Cherry Juice

This beverage is becoming more popular as the days go by. It is gotten from the fruit of the Prunus Cerasus tree. This juice is quite potent and offers a wide array of health benefits and nutrients to the body and it also helps in reducing symptoms of arthritis.

In a study conducted, 58 participants were given either a placebo or a 2 8-ounce bottles of tart cherry juice daily for 6 weeks. Participants that drank the tart cherry juice had a significant decrease in symptoms of osteoarthritis as well as reduced inflammation better than the people on placebo.

Another study showed that 20 women with osteoarthritis drank tart cherry juice for 3 weeks and experienced a reduction in the level of inflammatory markers.

Go for the unsweetened version to avoid you consuming excess added sugar. When you combine this in your diet with other arthritis fighting foods, a serving of unsweetened tart cherry juice daily would help to reduce some arthritis symptoms.

Foods to Avoid with Arthritis

Fried and processed foods

Researches from the Mount Sinai School of Medicine examined how to prevent diseases through one's diet. The study they carried out in 2009 showed that reducing the amount of processed and fried foods one eats can reduce inflammation and also restore natural defenses of the body.

What to do: reduce the amount of processed and fried foods you eat like store-bought prepared frozen meals and fried meats. Let your diet have more of fruits and vegetables.

Reduce your AGEs

This is an acronym for Advanced Glycation End product which is a toxin that appears when you heat, pasteurize, fry or grill foods. AGEs causes damage to certain proteins found in the body. In defense, the body attempts to break apart these AGEs by using cytokines which are messengers of inflammation. The side that the AGEs occurs would determine if it can lead to arthritis or other types of inflammation.

What to do: Research has proven that when you reduce the amount of foods that you cook at high temperature in your diet, it can in turn help to reduce the levels of blood AGE.

Sugars and refined carbs

When your diets contain high amounts of sugar, it can cause an increase in AGEs which would in turn cause inflammation.

What to do: cut out processed foods, candies, sodas and white flour baked goods to lower pain from arthritis.

Dairy products

Diary products contain protein that can add to arthritis pain. The protein may irritate the tissue around the joints for some people. However, a study done in 2017 claimed that anti-inflammatory properties can be gotten from milk except if the persons is allergic to cow milk. The available evidences are contradictory. If you are not sure how your body would react to diary, take it off your diet for about a month then reintroduce it to your diet and watch how your body would respond.

What to do: rather than getting your protein from dairy and meat, try getting from vegetables like nut butters, spinach, beans, quinoa and lentils to see if you would feel some improvement in your symptoms.

Alcohol and Tobacco

Using alcohol and tobacco can cause several problems with one's health including the ones that may affect the joints. If you are a smoker, you have a higher risk of developing rheumatoid arthritis while you have higher chances of getting gout when you consume alcohol too frequently.

What to do: to have healthy joints, you need a combination of physical activity, balanced diet and sufficient amount of rest, all of which can be compromised when you use tobacco and alcohol. I would advise that you cut back on smoking and drinking. Ensure that you include regular exercises, healthy meal choices and quality sleep in your daily sleep.

Salt and preservatives

Many foods that we eat have excess salt and other preservatives used to promote longer shelf lives. When you consume an excess amount of salt, it can cause inflammation of the joints. Reduce the quantity of salt that you take to as little as possible.

What to do: read labels and avoid foods with additives and preservatives. Less salts makes it easy to manage your arthritis and this includes not purchasing prepared meals. Although they are more convenient, however these prepared meals are usually very rich in sodium.

Corn oil

Several baked snacks and goods have corn or other oils that are rich in omega-6 fatty acids that can trigger inflammation. According to Mayo clinic, some studies showed that fish oil that has omega-3 can help in relieving joint pain.

What to do: rather than going for foods high in omega-6, replace them with healthy omega-3 alternatives like flax seeds, olive oil, pumpkin seeds and nuts.

Other foods you need to cut down on include:

- Red meat
- Dry roasted nuts and beer nuts
- Processed foods like prepackaged meals and commercial baked goods and bars.
- Certain oils like sunflower, peanut oils, corn, soy
- Refined grain products like white pasta and white bread

Achieving Results with the Anti-inflammatory Diet

While pain medications would require some few minutes to begin work, an anti-inflammatory diet on the other hand may not show any positive effects for days even up to several weeks. You may not be able to identify the effects as they come gradually, so I would advise that you keep a journal where you document changes in the symptoms that you experience. Even when you do not notice the difference in say a month or two, an anti-inflammatory diet has long term benefits as they help to reduce type 2 diabetes, heart disease and cancer.

It is important that you plan ahead before you begin the anti-inflammatory diet and choose a time where it would be easy for you to monitor and ensure success. You may want to begin your diet after a holiday or vacation where you would not be tempted with desserts and heavy foods. Once you get used to your new eating habits, it would then become easier to not to fall into temptations.

Anti-inflammatory Diet with Exercise
You can achieve far more pain relief when you combine the anti-inflammatory diet with routine exercise.

In one large study, pain and inflammation levels in patients with arthritis were compared between participants who were assigned to diet and exercise regimens and the ones assigned to diet or exercise. It was discovered that those who combined both exercise and diet benefitted more than the participants who were assigned to just exercise or just diet.

- The average pain levels reduced the most for people that combined exercise and diet.
- The people assigned to only healthy diet or exercise had about the same amount of reduced pain levels.
- Blood samples were used to measure inflammation levels and people who were assigned to combination of diet and exercise or just diet had the lowest levels.

Before you start an exercise routine with chronic arthritis or other medical conditions, it's important you consult with your doctor.

Impact of Weight on Arthritis

The most important connection between arthritis and your diet is your weight. Being overweight puts added strains on the joints that bears the body weight like your knees, ankles, back, feet and hips. Because of the way our joints function, the knee pressure is about 5 to 6 times your body weight when you walk so even the littlest of weight loss would make a great different. Also, when you have too much body fat, it would increase inflammation in the body which would cause the joints to be more painful. Researches have proven that when you lose excess weight, it can help to reduce inflammation no matter the type of arthritis you may have.

Guide to Lose Weight and Eat Healthy

Like we have said earlier on in this book, the only way you can lose weight and ensure that you do not gain such weight back is by changing the way you eat and the amount of exercise you do. Your food intake should be balanced with the amount of energy you burn. The energy in food is usually measured in kilocalories often called calories. If your meals have more calories than your body can use, your body automatically converts the extra calories to fat and you would notice that you begin to put on more weight. For some people, the more few extra calories they eat per day, the more weight they gain. For instance, if you consume 100 calories daily more than you burn off, it would add about 500g of fat to your body per month. However, if your food has lesser calories than your body needs, your body tends to burn stored up fat which would cause you to lose weight.

If you have been diagnosed with arthritis, it may be difficult to get as much exercise as before. And when you are not burning more energy, you are likely to put on excess weight except you reduce how much calories you consume. If you decide to reduce your calorie intake, it is important you keep a balance between the various kinds of food you eat so that you do not miss out on important nutrients. You need to consume starchy foods like rice, potatoes and pasta. The best options are the wholegrain types of pasta and rice as they have more fiber which is beneficial to the bowel while providing more minerals and nutrients. Vegetables and fruits (except fruit juices) are also low in calories but have plenty of beneficial nutrients.

Cut Down on Fats

Calories contained in fat are twice the amount that you have in protein or starch and most times, people tend to eat more fat than their body actually needs. When you eat 30 grams less fat daily, it would save you 270 calories.

There are four types of fats that can be found in foods:

Saturated fats: these are the most important types of fat that you need to reduce as they can cause an increase in inflammation and body pain. They are commonly gotten from animals and can be found in products below:

- Processed foods like biscuits cakes and pastry.
- Full fat diary products
- Asian foods particularly the ones cooked with ghee.
- Chips, when fried using animal fats.
- Some vegetable oils like coconut and palm oil.

Monounsaturated fats: these are neutral fats that can even be useful as they do not worsen inflammation. However, they have similar calories count as the saturated fats and it may be important to limit how you consume then when trying to lose weight. You can find them in rapeseed and olive oil.

Trans fats: these are the worst kinds of fat. They are gotten from chemically processed oil to make it solid and also increase shelf life. Not only do they increase cholesterol but are also dangerous to blood circulations and even your joints. When you check on the food label, you would see them listed as 'hydrogenated oil'.

Polyunsaturated oils:

- Omega-6 polyunsaturated fatty acids can cause an increase in inflammation in your body. Your aim therefore, should be to eat less of these softer fats and oils gotten from sunflower or corn.

- Omega-3 polyunsaturated fatty acids aver beneficial in the diet and can be found in walnuts, rapeseed oil, oily fish, free range eggs and fish oil supplements

If you want to eat less fats, you should:

- Avoid 'invisible 'fats in foods like cakes, biscuits, chocolate, savory snacks and pastry or limit their intake to special occasions.
- Go for olive oil, low fat or soya margarines.
- Go for lean cuts of meat and cut out any excess fat before you cook.
- Go for diary products that have low or reduced fats like low fat cheese or diet yogurt.
- Go for poultry and fish as often as possible.
- Grill rather than frying.

- make use of skimmed or semi skimmed milk.
- Make use of a little amount of olive oil for cooking if needed while you use rapeseed oil for frying food.
- Eat snacks that naturally have low fat like vegetable sticks, fruits and plain popcorn. Consuming nuts and seeds in small quantities help to provide good fat without causing weight gain.

Cut Down Your Sugar Intake

Sugar do not add any food value to our body as it only contains calories which is often called empty calories, so you are not losing any nutrients when you cut down on your sugar intake. When you eat 30 gram less sugar every day, it would save you approximately 120 calories.

Rather than using artificial sweeteners and sugar, why not go for dried fruits like raisins as sweetener for your puddings and cereals. Apart from helping to sweeten your meals, they would also provide minerals and vitamins. On the other hand, ensure not to overeat the dried fruits as they have fair amount of calories. The best option is to get used to eating your food without adding any sweetener or sugar.

Consume More Vegetables and Fruits

The World Health Organization (WHO) has advised that we need to consume at least 5 portions of vegetables and fruits each day, a portion is about 3oz. T

This would ensure that your body receives all the important nutrients that is needed for you to remain in good health and to protect you from the stress of diseases. Go for brighter colored veggies or salad to reduce your calorie intake while filling your plate.

Vegetables and fruits are rich in fibre and when you go for the ones with different colors, it would give you a vast options of minerals and vitamins. These bright colored veggies and fruits are packed with antioxidants like the leafy green veggies.

Exercise Regularly

Exercises would not only help to burn calories that would have turned into fat, but would also help to increase your suppleness and strength. However, if you have been diagnosed with arthritis, it may be quite hard and painful to exercise, so you would need to find an exercise that you can enjoy as this would be a motivating factor to get you to engage in it regularly. A good example is swimming which is very good for arthritis as it involves you moving all your muscles while the water helps to lift the weights from your joints. Other helpful exercises are yoga, Pilates and cycling.

Essential Minerals and Vitamins for Arthritis

Major part of the minerals and vitamins you need are gotten from the foods you eat rather than from supplements. If you do not get enough minerals and vitamins, it can make the arthritis to progress faster. The most important minerals and vitamins you need in treating arthritis are vitamin D, calcium and iron.

Vitamin D

Every person needs Vitamin D to maintain healthy and strong bones as well as other important roles that vitamin D plays to ensure that the body's health and wellbeing is improved. Your body needs Vitamin D to regulate and process the amount of phosphate and calcium within your body. These nutrients are helpful in developing your bone's structure and strength. If your body does not get the needed amount of Vitamin D, it can cause osteomalacia or osteoporosis.

Apart from being beneficial to the bone health, we need vitamin D for the following reasons:

- To boost your immune system (your body's way of fighting diseases)
- For healthy muscles.
- Lower your risk of having some types of cancer.

Vitamin D is often called the 'sunshine vitamin' because the best way you can get the vitamin is from the sun. When the sun gets to your skin, it allows the body to produce its own vitamins D. However, we cannot totally depend on sunlight to get all the vitamins D that our body need, all year round. Although we have foods that contain vitamin D, it may be difficult to get your body's daily amount from the foods you eat.

Because of the importance of vitamins D, we have been advised to consume vitamin D supplements for most part of the year at least. During winter and autumn, you should consider taking a 10 microgram of Vitamin D supplements daily. While we may have some people that can get enough vitamin D from combining healthy diet with sunlight, this is usually not so for everyone. If you belong to the group below, it is advisable that you take the vitamin D supplements all year round:

- People that wear clothes that cover the whole of the body and/ or face.
- People who do not go outside enough for example, those who live in a care home.
- Dark skinned people in ethnic minority groups. These includes people from Afro-Caribbean, African and South Asian backgrounds. This is because the dark skin pigmentation is not able to easily absorb vitamin D through the skin.

Vitamins D in Foods

Eggs and oil fish especially mackerel, salmon and herrings are foods that naturally have Vitamins D. Some foods are fortified with vitamins D like various breakfast cereals, margarine and powdered milk.

Is there an Excess of Vitamin D?

It can be harmful to consume more than 100 micrograms of Vitamin D daily as a supplement. For most people, it is sufficient for them to take a 10 micrograms Vitamin D supplement daily. If you keep overdosing on vitamins D gotten from supplements for a long period of time, it can cause a buildup of calcium in the body, a condition known as hypercalcemia. This condition can cause weak bone and is also bad for the kidneys and heart. If you have any worries, please reach out to your doctor for assistance.

On the other hand, it is not possible to get excess vitamins D from sunlight, but it's important to avoid being sunburned by ensuring that you are well covered if you have to stay out in the sunshine for a long time. Sunburn increases your risks of developing skin cancer in a later time.

Calcium

You need calcium to maintain healthy bones. When your body experience deficiency of calcium, it increases your risk of getting osteoporosis which can cause weakness in the insides of your bones and would put your bones at risk of breaking. This condition can commonly be seen amongst women that have passed menopause. You may also have a risk of having osteoporosis if you consistently take steroids on a long-term basis. Calcium deficiency can also increase your chances of developing osteomalacia, a condition that causes the outer shell of one's bones to go soft. This condition is also known as rickets

What are the best sources of Calcium?

They include

- Fish eaten with the bones like the tinned sardines.
- Calcium enriched milks made from oats, rice or soya
- Diary products like cheese, milk and yogurt. It's best to go for low fat ones and it makes no difference if they are from cows or other animals.

The skimmed and semi skimmed milk have more calcium than the full fat milk.

I would advise that you take 1,000 milligrams of calcium daily along with Vitamin D once you go past 60 years. If you are not able to eat as much diary products or foods rich in calcium, then you can take the calcium.

Recently, there has been concerns that if you take calcium supplements, it may impact negatively on the health of your heart. This concern applies only to calcium tablets and not the ones you get direct from foods. Increase the amount of calcium in your meal or discuss with your dietitian if you are worried.

Iron

Iron helps to prevent anemia which is a common condition in people that have arthritis. The two main causes are:

- Side effects of taking Nonsteroidal Anti-Inflammatory Drugs (NSAIDS) like ibuprofen, aspirin or diclofenac. Either you stop taking the NSAIDS or taking it along with another drug to protect the stomach would help to fix the anemia. You can also take iron supplements to replace the lost irons in the body caused by the NSAIDS.

- Anemia associated with chronic disease that often occur with rheumatoid arthritis and other similar conditions which do not improve even when you take iron supplements.

If you are anemic, consult your doctor to check if your condition can improve when you take more iron.

Good sources of iron include:

- Oily fish like sardines
- Red meat
- Dark green vegetables like kale, spinach and watercress.
- Pulses like haricots beans and lentils.

Your body is better able to absorb iron if taken with vitamin C, so it is advisable to add a portion of vegetables or fruits or a cup of fruit juice to your meal. It is also advisable not to drink tea while having your meal as it can reduce the amount of iron that your body can take at the time.

Vitamins C

Poor intake of vitamin C has been connected to arthritis. However, once you ensure that you have 5 portions of vegetables and fruits daily, you are not likely to have any problem with vitamin ac neither would you need supplements.

Fasting for Rheumatoid Arthritis

If you have the rheumatoid arthritis, fasting for short intervals can give a short-term improvement in the symptoms of this type of arthritis, although they are known to come back once you switch back to a normal diet. I would not recommend that you go on fasting to treat arthritis. However, if you want to try, it should be done under expert supervision and one day per time.

Food allergies

Several people are known to be allergic to some foods like shellfish or peanuts. These allergic reactions usually occur immediately you consume the food, however, there are still no scientific evidence to prove that food allergies are important in the development or treatment of arthritis.

Some people's body systems cannot tolerate some types of foods. The symptoms of these food intolerance slowly develop after you consume a food, from hours to as long as days. So, it can be very difficult to identify food tolerance without the help of experts.

Research has shown that some people may experience a positive progress in their symptoms when they avoid some types of foods. While we can't explain the reasons for this, the foods too also vary from person to person. Some diet books may also advise you to cut off important foods that would leave your body short of needed nutrients and minerals if you practice that diet for a long time. The only specific way to confirm food tolerance is by dietary 'exclusion and challenge' where you take out a certain food from your diet for a period, usually minimum of 1 month. Then you re-introduce the food to your diet to see if the food would cause any reaction to the body. If your arthritis is connected to food allergy you would notice that the symptoms would flare up within a few days of adding the new food. It is important that you totally cut out each food you wish to test and then re-introduce the foods one at a time. I would advise that you speak to a registered dietitian that would help to ensure that you are completely excluding foods and also check that you are not missing out on nutrients that the body needs.

Impacts of Vegan or Vegetarian Diet on Arthritis

From some studies conducted, it was shown that people that eat lots of red meat have a higher chance of developing inflammatory arthritis. Vegetarian diets have also been helpful over the years for several people that have the rheumatoid arthritis. A vegan diet that does not include fish, meat or other animal products may also be beneficial likely because of the polyunsaturated fatty acids that the diet has included.

If you go on the vegan diet, it is important that you make sure you get all the nutrients that you need especially calcium, vitamin D, B12 and selenium.

Calcium can be gotten from leafy green vegetables like kale, cabbage and broccoli, beans, watercress and chickpeas as well as some seeds, nuts and dried fruits. Also, calcium is usually added to white bread and some soya milk, rice milks and oats. It is important to read the food label.

Vitamin B12 can also be found in soya milk while another good source of vitamin B12 is the yeast extract.

Selenium can be gotten from nuts and often included in multivitamins supplements.

Vitamin D are not naturally found in many foods especially if you are on the vegan diet. However, you can naturally get it by exposing your body to sunlight. An alternative is to go for margarines and vegetable milks that have vitamin D added to them. Another source of the vitamin D is the shiitake mushrooms or you may have to go for supplements, there are available vegan supplements. Your aim should be 10 to 25 micrograms depending on how much you expose your skin to the sun.

Rewards of an Improved Lifestyle

An anti-inflammatory diet when combined with good sleep and exercise would provide you with several benefits some of which I would highlight below:

- Improvement in arthritis symptoms, lupus, inflammatory bowel syndrome and other autoimmune disorders.
- It would reduce inflammatory markers in your blood.
- Reduced risk of heart disease, obesity, cancer, diabetes, depression and other diseases.
- Improved mood and energy.
- Improved blood sugar, triglycerides and cholesterol levels.

Conclusion

While there are no specific arthritis diet plans as what works for you may not work for another person, but you can carry out trial and error to help you identify foods to remove from your diet. Most importantly, ensure to consume balanced diet and maintain a healthy body weight.

While we have some variety of foods that have powerful components to help provide relief from inflammation and arthritis, they would also help to provide your overall health.

When used alongside with conventional treatments, when you eat a nutritious diet that contains healthy fats, plenty of produce and a few servings of fatty fish, it would help to greatly relieve symptoms of arthritis.

Other Books by Nancy Peterson

- PREDIABETES ACTION PLAN AND COOKBOOK: Your Complete Guide to Reverse Prediabetes https://amzn.to/2YnAET0

- CELERY JUICE: The Natural Medicine for Healing Your Body and Weight Loss https://amzn.to/2xTTC4Z

- ENDOMORPH DIET PLAN: The Complete Guide to Loss that Excess Fat and Stay Healthy with Paleo Diet, Exercises and Trainings Perfect for Your Body Type. https://amzn.to/2xNU3NW

- The Diverticulitis Guide to Live Pain Free https://amzn.to/2JIdixY

- Apple Cider Vinegar: Your Complete Guide on How to Use https://amzn.to/2On99VX

- Cannabis cookbook https://amzn.to/2Ztq6Cfn

- Herbal medicines https://amzn.to/2Zjcevg

- Alkaline plant-based diet for beginners
  https://amzn.to/33ZVNTf

www.ingramcontent.com/pod-product-compliance
Lightning Source LLC
Chambersburg PA
CBHW051232250726
48655CB00006B/2723